The Stoic Body

How To Improve Your Health With Philosophy

ASHER BROCK

Contents

Introduction

The first known stoic was Zeno of Citium, who founded the idea in 301 BC. He took the name from Stoa Poikile, which translates to painted porch, and was a public market in Athens when the stoics met and discussed philosophy with anyone who wanted to learn. A second major figure of the early stoics was Crhysippus, who has been credited with elaborating the doctrine still associated with stoicism today. The early stoics were influenced by the previous philosophical thinkers and schools, especially Socrates and the Cynics, but also the Skeptics and Academics (the followers of Plato).

Next came the second period of stoic history, known as middle Stoa, which ushered in the philosophy to Rome. Cicero, a sympathizer to the stoic philosophy but not a stoic himself, is one of the major sources of the early and middle Stoa because only fragments of the writings of stoics exist up until that point. The third and final period of is referred to as late Stoa, and happened in the Imperial Rome time period. It includes the infamous stoics most people know about today, such as Gaius Musonius Rufus, Epictetus, Seneca, and Marcus Aurelius.

As Christianity blossomed and became the approved religion of Rome, stoicism began to decline, along with many other schools of thought. However, the idea of stoicism survived in many historical figures that were influenced by this line of thought, even though they were, at times, critical of stoicism. Some of the early Church Fathers, Thomas Aquinas, Boethius, Thomas More, Giordano Bruno, Montaigne, Erasmus, Descartes, Francis Bacon, Spinoza, and Montesquieu were influenced by stoicism. Modern neo-orthodox Protestants and modern Existentialism have both been influenced by stoicism. Recently, the philosophy as seen a rebirth, and has deeply influenced some modern practices such as cognitive behavior therapy and logo-therapy. It also has some similarities and overlaps with some modern philosophical approaches such as secular humanism and Buddhism.

There are eight important stoics you should know about before reading this book. Knowing a little about them and their beliefs is the glue that connects all of these practices together. The eight stoics are:

Zeno of Citium

Zeno was born around 334 BC and came from Cyprus, previously Citium, and was perhaps of Phoenician ancestry. He was the original forefather of stoicism, and educated others in Athens from around 300 BC until his death in 262 BC. Based on his moral ideas, stoicism had a high amount of importance on being good and having peace of mind, which was obtained from living a life in accordance of nature and virtue. It proved to be successful as a philosophy, and was the dominant philosophy from the Hellenistic time period during the Roman era.

Chrysippus of Soli

Chrysippus was born around 279 BC in Soli, Cilicia, but moved to Athens as a young man, where he decided to join a stoic school run by Cleanthes. When Cleanthes passed, around 230 BC, Chrysippus stepped in as the third head of the school. Chrysippus was a prolific writer who expanded the doctrines of Zeno of Citium, the founder of the original school. This earned him the title Second Founder of Stoicism.

Marcus Porcius Cato Uticensis

Marcus was born in 95 BC in Rome and is commonly known as Cato the Younger. Cato the Younger was known for his willfulness and persistence, especially during his conflict with Julius Caesar, as well as his moral integrity, immunity to bribes, and his distaste for the corruption of the time period. He passed away in April of 46 BC in Utica.

Porcia Catonis

Porcia Catonis was born around 70 BC and was the daughter of Atilia and Marcus Porcius Cato Uticencis. She was also known as Porcia the daughter of Cato and Portia in text, especially in the eighteenth century English literature. She's best recognized for being the second wife to Marcus Junius Uticenscis, the most prominent of Caesar's killers, and for his suicide, which was swallowing hot coals.

Lucius Annaeus Seneca

Often known just as Seneca, Lucius was born in 4 BC and was a statesman, Roman philosopher, humorist, and dramatist. In addition, he was an advisor and tutor to

Emperor Nero. Seneca was forced to commit suicide for his alleged complicity in the Pisonian conspiracy to kill Nero, but there is evidence he may have been innocent. His older brother was Lucius Junius Gallio Annaeanus, his father Seneca the Elder, and his nephew was Lucan the poet.

Gaius Musonius Rufus

Rufus was a roman philosopher of stoicism during the 1st Century CE. He taught philosophy in Rome while Nero was emperor, and was sent into exile in 65 CE as a consequence, but returned to Rome under Galba. When all other philosophers were banished from Rome in 71 CE, Rufus was allowed to stay, but he was banished later on, only to return after Vespasian, the emperor, died. A collection of extracts from what he wrote still survive today. He's also remembered as the teacher of Epictetus.

Epictetus

Epictetus was born in 55 CE and was a Greek philosopher born to a slave at Hierapolis, Phrygia, which is modern day Pamukkale, Turkey. He lived in Rome until he was banished, when he went to Nicopolis in Greece for the remainder of his days until 135 CE. His pupil, Arrian, wrote down and published Epictetus' writings in Discourses. Epictetus believed philosophy was more than just a theoretical discipline, but a way of life. To him, all external events were decided by fate, and are beyond control. We should accept whatever happens dispassionately and calmly. However, we're responsible for our own actions, which we can examine and control through self-discipline.

Marcus Aurelius

Perhaps the most infamous stoic of all is Marcus Aurelius , who was born on April 26, 121 and went on to become Emperor of Rome from 161 to 180. His co-emperor was Lucius Verus from 161 until Verus passed in 169. He was the final of the Five Good Emperors, and is thought of as one of the most significant stoic philosophers. His tome, Meditations, was written in Greek while he was on campaign during 170 and 180, and is still admired as a literary tribute to philosophy.

Now that you're aware of the basic history of Stoicism, let's take a look at the philosophy and how it can be applied to modern-day living.

Chapter One – Understand Your Life's Purpose

The first lesson to be learned from Stoicism is the foundation of Stoicism – understanding your life's purpose and living life on purpose. If you don't know at the core what you want to do with your life, a thousand other things will rush in and take over. At the end of your life, you'll see that you lived other people's demands and interests rather than yours. You need to own your days so they do not own you. The first way to practice this is to start with a morning routine.

Morning Routine

The alarm goes off, and you have exactly one hour to be out your door. After you finally stop hitting the snooze button and spend a few minutes looking at your phone, you get up. You put together your coffee, feed pets, get your kids together, and help someone get something to eat. In ten minutes, the disorder of the a.m. urgency has taken over everything, in addition to that niggling feeling that you have some messages to send out before you head for that meeting at work. So much for easing into your day peacefully.

Even if you have a partner and use a tag team approach, it's still a major production to get into the shower and get ready for work. There are bags that need packed, homework to be gathered, bills to be paid, and goodbyes to be said as everyone goes out the front door.

Once you get to work, it's a dash to get things done before that morning meeting. Somehow, you wait for a quiet moment in order to pull together your final thoughts, to breathe or catch up, but that chance distances itself further and further. Later, you think maybe you can get some time at lunch, or after work, or at night, and then you're collapsing into bed only to wake up to the blaring alarm clock again.

That's the first scenario – the one where you don't have a morning routine. If you're like most people, this is you. However, let's look at how it *can* be.

The second scenario is the alarm goes off. This time, you have about two and a half hours. There's no snooze button during this scenario. Before anyone else in the household gets up, you get your ready-made coffee thanks to your pre-programmed coffee machine and slip into a remote area of the house where everything you need for your morning routine is set up. Your phone is upstairs because it's only there if you need it to wake you up. After you journal or read for a few minutes while you sip your coffee, you do a little meditation, yoga, or stretching to get ready for your morning workout. You enjoy the quiet surrounding you and focus on your movements. While you take some time afterward, you write out the main list for what you'll get done that day. After a shower, you're feeling peaceful and prepared to wake up the rest of the family and face the day.

Direct, or you're going to be put in a constant position of reacting.

While few people get to choose what happens during their day, the morning has the power to determine what or who is going to be leading the way and how much we give to our interests versus responding to someone else's as the day goes on. Your willpower is at its best in the morning, before you've had to fend off the slew of choices and issues that come your way. In other words, if you have a hard time keeping a commitment to yourself, you'll most likely be more successful making it part of the morning routine rather than holding off until later during the day.

From a psychological viewpoint, the morning hours offer some extra benefits. Exercising when you've fasted offers you greater benefits for insulin sensitivity and fat burning. There's the advantage of having that morning cortisol burst, too. This means extra energy that will go a long way in a morning exercise routine or to help you tackle your more challenging tasks. How many people postpone their exercise and responsibilities as long as possible, only to have to face them throughout the least active and driven hours in your day? By this point, it takes ten times the mental and physical capacity to make yourself follow through.

Another benefit is that you're more devoted to making healthier decisions during the day if you've already worked out in the morning, meditated, and performed other positive actions. You've previously invested in living a healthier lifestyle. You won't be subject to the troublesome sense of anxiety that follows you everywhere during the day. Your body is waiting to move and ready to protest at having to sit at a desk for eight hours.

People like to call their deferment of meditation and exercise as being self-discipline, but really, it's self-deprivation.

Developing a morning routine will let you assert your authority over the day. You take charge of your work-life equilibrium by paying yourself first, in a sense. Too many people do it the other way around and are left without enough time and energy to invest in themselves at the end of the day. As a result, many people feel they are at the mercy of their family and work demands. Responsibilities overwhelm them, and they end up getting stuck.

If you lead with your peace and well-being in the morning, however, you can get a lot more done during the day. Something essential will change when you start directing your day instead of responding to it. However you decide to design your morning routine, you're claiming the day before anyone or anything else is able to. Your actions, and the pattern of that action over time, will create a strong shift in your personal sense of fulfillment and happiness.

If you can't think of anything to start your day off with, let me help you.

Physical Health

The first thing people think of when they think of doing a physically healthy routine in the morning is exercise, but with that said, there are some other things that can help you physically in the morning. Make sure to go outside because the light can help you naturally wake up, and you'll feel more awake if you get in a good morning run or walk if it's outside. In addition, keep in mind that you don't have to move your whole workout routine to the morning if that doesn't work for you. Do a short stroll in the morning and save the rest for later. The idea is to do some kind of movement, like walking, yoga, or lifting a few weights, in addition to what else you feel would fuel your physical health for the day.

Mental Health

Your mind is just as important as the rest of your body. Yoga might do it for you, or a little time outside. Some people like to have their breakfast or coffee outside, and just that little action makes a huge difference for the day.

Other people like to meditate from five to thirty minutes, and some like to read a book or write in a journal to center themselves. Others use the time to indulge in a little self-care.

Personal Vision

Your morning routine should have something that pertains to your personal vision. This is important because it relates to the direct-react problem in a larger way than just one day's agenda. Many of us have greater visualizations for our lives, such as things we want to try, careers we want to get into, hobbies we want to enjoy, or ideas they want to study, but they never do. If you're waiting until nine at night or a 'free' weekend, you can file that under the 'it's never going to happen' drawer.

Be brave, give a portion of your day's best energy to your vision, and maybe you'll learn a new hobby or get into a new career. Perhaps it's fitness, or it's a creative adventure. Maybe you want to network and build your portfolio to shift your career. Whatever it is, start your day off with it. If you stick with this one action every morning, you'll be amazed at your progress in just a few weeks, months, and over the time span of a year.

Do Something Productive

Like with any of the aforementioned ideas, this can mean something different for each person. Make a master list for your day, as a suggestion. You don't need to write down fifty things on a piece of paper. Just put down five of the most important ones, and make sure you do the most important and challenging ones first thing in the morning. Beyond this, you could do a chore that will make a difference in the following few days ahead. Devote a few hours to some financial planning or record keeping for the next week.

Experiment

Morning routines are *your* time, so it should be time that is yours and involves no one else. Lock the door if you have to. So few people are accustomed to giving themselves this much-needed time. Putting yourself first during the morning can feel a little weird. You may be overwhelmed by how much you want to do in the morning, or you might not know how to fill the space. Just choose one thing at a time and build on the routine. If you stick with it and use it to benefit you, then you'll wonder how you ever lived without one.

Meditating on Your Life's Purpose

1. Start with one area of your life in mind. Choose an area where you're struggling or you want to experience a transformation, such as your career, your relationship with your spouse, or a hobby you want to turn into a business.

2. Begin to imagine the highest outcome you want to be living in from six to twelve months from this moment in this area of your life. Imagine living your life the way you want with all your hope and dreams coming true. What is the reality? Try not to get hung up on limitation or negativity. Just let yourself get carried away with the wildest aspirations you can imagine.

3. Connect with a single goal you want to achieve in the following three months. If you choose a goal without a lot of meaning or weight, the end result is not going to feel that special. So be sure to choose something that's large enough that, once

you achieve this goal, you'll feel accomplished and motivated to set another goal.

4. Now that you've connected with the goal, imagine your life once you've completed the goal. Make a mental movie or picture in your mind and step inside that visual representation.

5. Step outside of your image and imagine floating up above where you're at now, taking that mental image with you. Inhale deeply, and as you exhale, use your breath to energize that image, filling it with intention and positive energy. Do this a total of five times.

6. Imagine floating into the future and visualize dropping that internal representation of your goal down into your life at the date and time you set for when the goal should be completed.

7. Notice how the events between your current reality and future reality support you in realizing your objective.

8. Once you feel you've finished, return to reality, and as you keep your eyes closed, consider the action steps you need to take in the next week to move closer to the goal.

9. Breathe deeply in order to make yourself feel centered before you open your eyes. Jot down the list of action steps you need to take.

10. Keep your focus and take action. Each day, take an action step that gets you closer to achieving your goal.

Chapter Two - Create a Gratitude Record

Any type of gratitude practice can benefit you. Some people like to do a meditation every day, while others like to write in a journal. In the future, having a gratitude journal means you can look back at the positive situations you've appreciated and the positive outlook you had whether a day was bad or good. You're reminded life is made up of both negative and positive occasions, and as stoics like to say, you can maintain the most tranquility when you attach yourself to neither but spot the inescapable pendulum at work.

This raises the issue of what you'll put in your journal. Some people complain it's just going to end up being the same stuff on a daily basis, such as their job, children, and food. And yes, these are all legitimate things to put in the journal, but look a little closer for other things. Were you fortunate today? Did you do something well? Did something go as you planned? What did you learn when something bad happened? How did life appear to you today? What did you see in your kids? What things did you appreciate about your spouse? Did someone compliment you today? What did you get the chance to observe today that inspired you?

If you're having a hard time finding something to be grateful for every day, then it's probably because you're not taking the opportunity to really look at what you come across.

Let's take a look at an example of something you can be grateful for.

Gratitude about Health

Think about the last time you had a major illness, be it the flu, a cold, food poisoning, or something similar. Think about how awful you felt - the puffy, burning eyes, terrible headache, and the clogged sinuses. During the illness, you probably couldn't imagine what it was like to be healthy again. You could barely remember what life was like three days prior when you were taking care of the kids, getting work done, and exercising. Fast forward, and you're dealing with mental fatigue and physical misery. This is just the flu or a cold. Many people have it a lot worse. However, it's a relatable illustration of a common truth —

people tend to take their health for granted until it's just gone one morning.

Three days before, you might have felt good about your workout performance, or finished it off begrudgingly. You might have gotten out of bed realizing you had a good night's rest, or you were too lost in the negative anticipation of the day to let yourself feel well. You might have treasured having the vigor you needed to keep up with your children, or felt preoccupied by stress and expended a lot of time managing your world on your phone or running through an imagined conversation with your boss. In a normal day, you barely notice your health, unless its limitations disrupt your routine or intentions.

It means a lot to be grateful for your health. At the most basic level, it can be a feeling you get when someone you know passes of a heart attack or is diagnosed with cancer. The news jolts you to the awareness of your mortality, with your health being what keeps you going.

However, being thankful for your health is more than just being grateful for being alive. On another level, it translates to being thankful for your overall health and the capacities you have, such as the cognitive capability to practice your occupation and recollect your kids' names, or the physical capability to walk up five flights when the elevator is serviced. It's the security of understanding you can travel to a remote place and deal with whatever conditions you come across. It's the freedom to go skiing and attempt something new minus getting enveloped in the fear of being frail. It's about the confidence and strength to move things on your own when the need comes about.

Everyone receives something good each day. Traditional societies were a little more in touch with this sense of being a recipient of something when they were alive. Modern individuals are inclined to believe they make everything occur on their own, and this attitude undercuts the gratitude. It's why those who go through tough periods are a little more grateful for the good times. They've faced losses and events that others cannot imagine, and the small things seem to be magnified. When you live each day in the present moment because you choose to or because you need to, you are not as likely to dismiss the positive things.

A gratitude journal is one of the things that pays off the longer you do it. Don't worry if it feels stupid or forced in the beginning. This is for no one but you. You'd be surprised by how deeply a gratitude journal will change your outlook on life and how that shift will cause deep changes.

Chapter Three - Have Boundaries

Boundaries are not enclosures or walls. The idea is not to isolate yourself or refuse to live in a community with others or collaborate with those around you. Having boundaries is about acknowledging that you're working with some limited resources – energy and time. To pretend you're not limited in these resources is a delusion.

Try to think of living with boundaries are managing an investment. If you give all your energy and time away to unhelpful emotions and negative thoughts, such as worry, anger, and guilt, then you'll have nothing left for the overall purpose of your life and the people who are living it with you. Perhaps ancient people didn't have to worry about a central vision, but they also didn't need to sort through the million tasks, inputs, and notifications modern people do on a daily basis. If it's a contest of who is at risk of not living life, then it's the modern humans.

Think about what endeavors and relationships sustain your will to go on, foster your good health, and serve your overall vision of life. Invest in these relationships and actions. Let the rest go, or at least budget the amount of time you spend thinking about it. There is nothing wrong with being selective. No person should or can be responsible for everyone and everything that happens in life. To be a useful presence in the here and now, you have to be a balanced person. You can't sustain or become that by being at the whim of someone else's demands, suggestions, or judgements.

Behind all good intentions – the short-term strategies, overall goal, and daily routines – is the bottom line. What's the least you're willing to accept from yourself on any given day? This question is the most important one you will ever ask yourself.

The biggest obstacle most people have is their perception of their circumstances, time, bodies, and potential. Anyone can create a goal, but it's how they weave their intentions into their daily reality that gets them to the finish line.

People go through their daily lives thinking their intentions are important but negotiable. At the same time, they unconsciously or consciously view other's intentions for them as fixed, or non-negotiable. This is where the method fails.

If you're daily objectives are negotiable, then they're disposable.

Yes, everyone has a life with components. Your job takes you past your regular quitting time or calls for you to travel. The children fall ill or your babysitter does. Finances are tight. The weather sucks. The car is broken. And you get low on enthusiasm and steam. You hit period of major transition in your life that are sparked in a moment, but they're drug on for months.

These facts are never going to change. Life is always going to fluctuate. If you wait to start a health commitment until things 'settle down', then you'll be sitting on the curb forever. If you tell yourself you won't have to negotiate away your intended actions when you have an easier week, you'll forgo progress. Reality dictates circumstances are going to take your time. People are going to ask things of you at the last minute. Your energy is going to feel depleted before you have finished your priorities. And there's where you decide if it's up to you to let go of something you had planned for yourself.

Life requires flexibility of you, to an extent. If you hang onto predictability too much, then you'll make yourself or everyone around you miserable or you'll diminish your life down to nothing. In addition, there are times when missing your exercises, or going light on yourself, is the best choice for you.

However, you can choose to draw the line in the sand when it's important.

What this means is there are non-negotiable rules you under no circumstances break. There is one thing you do on a daily basis that you do for you, no matter what. If you don't take a firm stake for that one thing, life is going to take it from you.

Non-negotiable rules ought to be practices that you commit to on a daily basis, no matter what. This is something that you will never go a day without doing.

The key to creating a non-negotiable rule is to envision a single objective you'll fulfill on a daily basis without any excuses. Think of it as a mantra to live by. Either way, it'll keep you directed toward your health daily.

For example, a fitness guru might say they will never go a day without sweating.

A yoga person might say they will never go a day without doing at least one yoga move.

It might be something as simple as saying you will always go to bed at or before nine at night.

If you feel you have to see your non-negotiable commitment in a different way, you could decide you will never skip a gym workout on Tuesdays and Thursdays. Even if you adjust the workout, you'll get to the gym on those days.

If your focus is on dieting now, then you could commit to eating a certain amount of fat or protein or carbohydrates every day.

Another choice that pertains to food would be to intermittently fast for a portion of each day, or a set number of days a week, even if you decide you won't eat anything after six at night.

The idea of these rules is multi-dimensional. Yes, you get an obvious benefit of doing something healthy every day, and you create a fixed, real cornerstone for your health commitment. In this sense, you will never completely abandon your vision. Each day you take a step to thrive. However, you'll benefit from the impact of association. One positive choice daily will empower another positive choice.

If you know you're going to be doing one healthy action for yourself, especially if you do it during your morning routine, then you'll automatically support a perception of your day and yourself. For example, you've made the decision to be grateful in the morning, which means you might make the decision to be positive and consciously grateful throughout the day.

The example I just mentioned might seem simple and elementary, and if they are, then make your non-negotiables a little more ambitious, but remember this is your bottom line, not the upper limit. Making a non-negotiable commitment doesn't keep you from being better in the future; it's just a bottom line limit you will accept of yourself. In fact, you should aim to do better than your non-negotiables each day, but start with them.

In addition, your non-negotiable action should and ought to change. You might say you will start going to bed at eleven at night, but then realize that you need to get in a little more sleep, so you change your non-negotiable to ten. You may decide that it's become easy to count the protein in your diet, so you move on to counting both protein *and* fat. Or you might decide that you can do more than just be grateful in the morning, you can move on to do something someone else will appreciate, too.

The ultimate goal of your non-negotiable is the practice itself. When you get better at seeing your goals as essential and important, and other demands on your time are negotiable, then you will come to value the commitment to your life. Likewise, the more creatively you will change to fill your other obligations in different ways.

You'll use your time and energy better, knowing you have to save something for your non-negotiable goals. You'll assess the time you're spending with your friends and family and ask if you're prioritizing the experiences that mean the most and draw you closer to them. You'll begin to think about what really helps you make quality relationships and work, as well as how you can foster the health that lets you give the most to these individuals and your life goals over time.

Chapter Four – Make a Detachment Practice

This is the other side of keeping a gratitude record, but it create gratitude in a way. The idea of this chapter is to teach you to let go of attachment in your life, such as attachments to the outcomes you want, attachments to the conditions you feel are important, attachments to your possessions, and attachments to the relationships you feel you can't live without.

On one side, there are the small things, such as the outcomes you desire and just the small things you want in life. It's important to understand that life is good even if you don't get everything you want. Someone once said that 'as long as everything is exactly how they want it to be, then they are completely flexible.' It's meant to be funny, but the truth is that there are people who actually live their lives this way. Life is going to be challenging enough. You don't need to set yourself up for a greater challenge by fueling your expectations or living rigidly. Sometimes, not getting what you desire is one of the greatest things possible.

Letting Go of Expectations

Something many successful individuals say is that you need to be focused, but if you ask them to elaborate, they will tell you that it's not others you have to be focused on but yourself. That doesn't mean you shouldn't be aware of the people around you, but that you cannot afford to spend your energy outside of yourself when you're trying to accomplish something. You can't afford to waste your critical mental resources.

Focusing on other people and getting diverted through the comparison trap is a perilous mistake. Your success is not about where other people are in their lives. It's about your focus and state of mind. Some people can come with a strategy they've established over weeks but get flung off course by putting too much weight on what others are doing. All of a sudden, they've put so much energy on focusing on others than on themselves that they've lost their way. They struggle to catch up to their goals. There is a time and place for comparison, but you need to be mindful when you're comparing and what you're looking to obtain from it.

There is an important factor here. When you're learning with others, offering mutual encouragement to each other, is community. There's something to the group dynamic when it comes to learning. The energy and presence of others who want to succeed can help you move forward, too. They can help you make light of a difficult task. They can offer you support. They can share the emotional and physical journey with you. Having a witness to struggles and accomplishments is a powerful thing.

However, setting their capabilities and performance against your own, is comparison. The first doesn't always lead to the second, but it can accompany it. The same is true for numerous situations, whether you're getting into shape, losing weight, rebuilding health, growing your finances, or growing your career. How you handle your inclination toward community and comparison is up to you.

The Benefit of Comparison

The social comparison theory tells us that we compare ourselves to others for information gathering purposes, or as a means for honing or expanding our frame of reference for self-assessment. There's a reality check when unbiased methods are not there or are not deemed as being applicable. In some cases, we'll liken ourselves to others because we wish to motivate ourselves to obtain more by finding motivations in the examples of upward evaluation, such as someone who is fitter, more successful, or just happier. In other circumstances, we'll choose to indulge in downward comparison to boost our self-esteem by focusing on those who are in worse situations than ours, such as those who are less fit, less successful, or just overall less happy.

On the positive end of the spectrum, comparison offers you an information gathering point of reference. You might not realize what's possible without taking a look at others. The example of someone else can expand your sense of what you can do. Perhaps you never understood the different approaches to getting healthy or preparing your own meals. Maybe you never believed it was possible to work at home or balance the need between personal time and family commitment. In addition, seeing the struggles and successes of others can help you anticipate the troubles and find the right solutions for your own adventures.

However, these examples are the more harmless ones that fall more under an observation ritual than true comparison.

When it comes to true assessment-focused comparison to others as people usually think of it, the impact of their behavior is varied but clear. Studies have shown that people tend to use others in their inner circles as the norms against which they gauge their eating habits and overall weight. Using that idea, you can feel genuinely motivated to do better. Research has shown that people increase their efforts solely based on their perception of the person who is exercising next to them. One of your inclinations is to push yourself or slack off depending on who is around you. Experts believe that comparing some part of yourself can support self-enhancement and self-esteem.

It's the age-old adage of surrounding yourself with positive influences in order to get more done.

The Downside of Comparison

However, not every comparison is a good one. While research in the area of social comparison has shown that people tend to compare themselves to others who are more similar instead of vastly different in characteristics, capabilities, and other aspects available for evaluation, people tend to look for the comparison they're trained to seek out, whether it's by their emotional insecurities or modern media's influence. How many times have you seen photos of a really great looking model and wondered why you can't look like that? How many times have you slunk to the other side of the gym so you're not standing next to the most muscular guy or gal in the room?

On the flipside, maybe you've taken some steps to eat better and not felt motivated to continue forward because your choices are so much better than those of the people in your family or social circle. It's too easy to feel good about a few small steps when almost everyone you know is so far behind you already.

You need to be completely honest and mindful about the motivation behind your comparison. What are you really looking at when you're looking at everyone else at the gym? What's really going through your head when you go for the front or back row of the fitness class? What are you looking to see in those around you? Are you gathering information on ideas and techniques? Or are you looking for ammunition to use against yourself to affirm some rooted thought processes, or for justification to boost your ego?

There is nothing wrong with asking a legitimate question that leads you toward a more productive self. How is that person pacing their workout? Do they enjoy training? Is that person more successful at sales because of how they behave? What did that person do in order to get into the position they are in the business?

The next question that should come to you after those types of questions is, 'Why not me?'

Healthy comparison ought to bring you back to empowerment. Marcus Aurelius stated that, "How much time he gains who does not look to see what his neighbor says or does or thinks, but only at what he does himself…"

Every five minutes you spend on comparing your capabilities to someone else, you should spend an hour assessing your progress and doing something to celebrate it. You're your ultimate frame of reference. Keep track of whatever you have to in order to measure your self-comparison. Keep your mind on your progress. Hone your performance by knowing and following what demonstrates to you your progress.

Make sure to be honest with yourself about what is giving you a positive input for consideration and what will push you too far right now. Your confidence will grow as your self-investment increases and your skills increase. You don't have to have everything perfect as soon as you begin. Stay away from media that's sending you down negative comparison paths. Be mindful with settings that might trigger your insecurity, but don't use it as an excuse to avoid resources that are helpful to your goals.

You have to commit to seeing yourself in a better light. Don't be your own worst critic and engage in excuses, self-bashing, and victimhood. No matter what everyone else around you is doing, it won't matter more than your attitude toward yourself does.

Lastly, lean on a like-minded community and be sure you're not going it alone. Community supports instead of compares. Isolation will breed comparison. When you feel you're connected with others, you'll feel more secure. When you're supported and known, it's not about comparing yourself to others with arrogance or envy. It's about being known and knowing you're a fallible, aspiring person.

Yes, when it comes down to the deeper things in life, such as your relationships, it's a little harder. As much as you might like to think otherwise, nothing is permanent. No one is guaranteed anything in life except the end of it. Instead of getting depressed about this eventuality, you can embrace it and see it as a reason to hold your possessions and connections lightly. You can care about them and enjoy them without identify all of life or happiness with them. It doesn't mean you can't love someone, a pet, or something with all your heart, but know that it is not a given.

That is how detachment breeds gratitude. You can be grateful for what you have now, and know that it will not last forever.

Chapter Five – Create a Resilience Plan

Humans have it easier than we used to. With our climate controlled homes, advanced outdoor clothing, public and private transit, shopping, indoor plumbing, and delivery, it's entirely doable for us to live life without having to walk too far, lift too much, shiver a little, sweat, or otherwise be in tune with what's 'hard' about having a physical body. Our ancestors lived with variability in a way that most people are cut off from now. You'd have to live in a third world country to understand what it was like to live during ancient history. Reapplying that into our lives with cold water therapy, imposed power outages, and other physical measures can help your body and mind recalibrate to a more resilient and flexible center.

Similarly, getting out of your comfort zone and doing something that allows to see the aspects of community and life you'd like to pretend doesn't exist can help you get in touch with a truth larger than yours and help you build mental strength, as well as emotional resilience.

Build Mental Fortitude

It's in the resolve that's seen in physical therapy patients who are told they will never walk again, only to go to physical therapy every day of the week and do what it takes to prove doctors wrong. It's in the homeless individual who still manages to scrape together enough to take care of someone else, whether it's a friend or pet. It's in the overweight individual who manages to shed the pounds all the way down to their goal weight, and then some.

Resilience can contain the physical and emotional stamina you need to get through a few rough weeks or bounce back from an injury or illness. However, even more important, resilience can mean the fortitude to handle life-changing events, and even grow from them.

Resilience is not a superhero trait. People talk about conquering their limitations, overcoming their loss, and beating back illnesses; however, the reality is a little more complex than that. Those clients and friends who have been models of resilience have been completely human at some point. Not every day is going to be a good day for them. Not every step will lead them forward.

The man who cares for someone else despite being homeless may have breakdowns as he tries to figure out how to make money. The woman who lost all that weight, and then some, broke down and ate things she shouldn't have or neglected to exercise for a week because she just wanted to give up. The person who was told they would never walk again may have had a moment of defeat before going to those physical therapy classes.

Everyone has to pick themselves up at some point, and some days, you'll let yourself down a little longer than others. You feel what you have to feel. The pivotal point is recovering and reengaging in life on renewed terms.

Psychologists have taken a look at this phenomenon known as resilience and determined it is a varying characteristics amongst people. Some, when they're faced with hardship, are buoyed by a sense of energy and perspective. They're more likely to get back to life while others struggle a little more. Resilience appears to be a trait that's influenced by our brains, or the molecular operations that process stress.

However, it's a mindset that is able to be nurtured into a flexibility to handle the rough times in life, as well as the willingness to live with the unknown. Research has demonstrated that the more resilient we are, the more satisfaction we obtain from life.

There are a few different ways you can cultivate resilience in your life.

Exercise

A solid foundation for your health with all the basics covered will help you with any of the stoic beliefs in this book. Diet, sleep, and getting enough movement are all important when it comes to being resilient. However, some research has shown that exercise may be a little more important that the others. Stress, anxiety, depression are all being fought with exercise. When compared with the rest, a thirty-minute block of moderate exercise is better at decreasing anxiety when individuals are exposed to photographs with stress-inducing images.

However, exercise cannot be performed once and you expect to see results. You have to stick with a routine of exercise in order to see some long-term impact. Regular exercise will create a continuing psychological difference that changes your stress response. Over time, exercise will contribute to your mental resilience.

Mindfulness

In the middle of a major life change, you can benefit from the nostalgia of envisioning future endeavors. However, what's also important is the capability to be completely in the moment, to release your questions, expectations, and plans. Mindfulness, in addition to eliciting the body's relaxation response, has a major role in acceptance, a crucial process for living with a challenging situation.

People tend to expend a lot of energy and worry pushing back against a difficult challenge when they'd be better off shifting gears and realigning themselves with their new reality. Similarly, it can take a lot of patience to handle an emotion. There are things people unnecessarily accept when they have an opportunity to change the situation. However, there is a difference between conscious acceptance and resignation. If you talk to the survivor of a major crash, they'll tell you acceptance isn't a passive undertaking. It's a growing, dynamic, and ongoing process. True mindfulness with help with this process.

Mindfulness will take on a different meaning for each person. Some might practice Tai Chi, yoga, or some other type of passive exercise. Others might want to immerse themselves in a meaningful ritual or pray. And some might seek peace just by spending time in nature, allowing their involuntary attention to take over their mind, allowing them to let go of everything but the awareness of what's happening around them.

Social Connection

One of the main things we all need, as humans, is a social connection with others. That doesn't mean you need three hundred friends on Facebook, or even three friends. It means you need to have as many friends as it takes to make you feel socially connected, and that could be just one person.

Everyone knows how good it feels to have a shoulder to lean on when they're not feeling up to par or times are tough. A strong support system can be there to provide you with the logistical and emotional help you need when you're going through a challenge, but close friends and family can make a difference in how you handle the challenges of normal life changes. Close friendships are one of the most key influences on how you adapt to life in your later years. Overall, your close social connections might dampen the stress of these normal experiences by giving you the important outlet you need for the different emotions life will evoke, and they can provide you with perspective when you see your friends going through these struggles of their own.

Play

Take a moment to watch some kids play at the playground, or spend a day with one of your young nephews, nieces, or cousins if you don't have kids of your own to watch. Observe how children play in order to experiment with a different variety of emotions, ideas, and experiences they come across in their development. Children go through play therapy when they're processing a transition, trauma, or another type of difficult event. Across experience and lifespan, play creates connections and encourages behavioral, emotional, and intellectual flexibility.

Humans maintain the capacity to play throughout their lifetimes, and for a good reason. As a result of playing, the exploration, experimentation, and creativity it encourages, you can continually change to fit with different circumstances. When you expand yourself beyond the daily practice of specialization and efficiency, you can see yourself and life with a fresh pair of eyes. Play makes you intellectually and emotionally stronger.

For adults, play might mean anything from participating in a competitive sport to finding a creative endeavor. Many people take up different hobbies after a severely stressful event, such as the death of a loved one or a divorce. The hobbies give these people a sense that there is something new for them in the future. Play, however it comes about, it an experimental space where you can find emotional peace.

No one knows what their life will look like. Amidst many joys, there are going to be troubles. Some problems will just crop up suddenly, and others we'll make for ourselves.

Regardless of where they come from, we'll struggle against failure, illness, change, and loss. Many have already navigated some critical transitions in their lives.

When our ancestors were alive, troubles were much more frequent. Our ancestors weren't as consumed by the smaller stresses of life because death and danger were always around the corner, especially in a way most people are not used to in modern life. What supported our resiliency and physical survival then can serve our psychological resilience today – mental flexibility, social connectedness, intellectual creativity, and emotional balance.

Resiliency is not a fixed ability, and it's not in indefinite supply. You'll continually make and remake your resilience by investing in your engagement with others and with life. Your daily connections and practices over time will deepen your resilience. What helps you thrive right now will grant you with fortitude for the future.

Mindfulness Meditation

1. Take a seat. Whatever you're sitting on – bench, chair, cushion, or a blanket – find a spot that makes

you feel stable and solid rather than hanging back or perching.

2. Notice how your legs are. If you're on a cushion, cross your legs in front of you. If you're doing a yoga pose, continue. If you're on a chair, put the bottoms of your feet on the floor.

3. Straighten your upper body but make sure not to be stiff. The spine has a natural curve. Let it curve naturally.

4. Place your upper arms parallel with your upper body. Allow your hands to drop to the tops of your thighs. With your arms at your side, your hands will naturally fall to the right location.

5. Drop your chin a bit and allow your vision to fall downward gently. You might let your eyelids lower. If you feel the need, then close them completely, but you don't have to.

6. Be in this spot for a few moments. Breathe and relax. Bring your attention to the sensations in your body.

7. Feel your breath as it's going in and out of your body. Draw your attention to the physical feeling of breathing.

8. Your attention will wander to other things than your breathing, but don't worry. There's no need to eliminate or block your thoughts. As you get around to your mind drifting, softly return your thoughts to your breath.

9. Pause before you make any physical adjustments, like moving your body or scratching something. Shift your body with intention, allowing the space between what you experience and what your next action is.

10. You might find your mind is wandering all the time. This is normal. Rather than engaging or wrestling with your thoughts, practicing observing without needing to react to them. Pay attention and do nothing.

11. When you're ready, lift your vision or open your eyes. Take a moment to notice sounds in your environment. Notice how you feel right now. Notice your emotions, thoughts, and physical body. Pause momentarily and decide you want to proceed with your day.

Chapter Six - Understand What You Have Control Over

The original descriptions for what we have control over by the stoics were 'what we have no control over' and 'what we have complete control over'. However, there is a third category; the things we have partial control over.

In the moment of trying to figure out a solution to a problem, it's easy to believe we have complete control over every facet of an issue. A fantasy crops up that tells us we better make something happen or get a handle on the situation immediately. However, it's time to unclench your jaws and allow your tightened fists to slacken a little, and get a real grip on what you can and cannot do.

Breathe for a moment and get out a piece of paper. Across the top of the page, write down what you have complete control over, what you have some control over, and what you have no control over. It's an instant perspective if you're honest with yourself.

Don't think of this as just a useful practice on occasion. You should do this with every significant problem you have in your life. The benefit of doing this will make you more efficient at applying your emotional investment and logistical efforts. A good leader will apply themselves efficiently.

Self-Control

Many stoics edit their environment as they practice. They may work from home and have their favorite places to go, as well as a close circle of like-minded friends and family. The nature of their work will put them in contact with those who have similar goals to them. Even their media might be customized. Without thinking about it, their environments will become stoic-oriented.

However, when you go out, it might feel a little like a culture shock. For example, let's say you go to a movie theater. Have you ever noticed that when an ad comes on the screen for soda, people will drink their sodas? Or when popcorn or candy is on the screen, they'll eat their choice of movie-going snack. People feel an emotional affirmation around their decision to purchase all the junk food they did when they see someone else affirming it's a good choice.

In a culture where we worship impulse, self-control doesn't have a lot of appeal. Think about it. We all want to eat a cookie over that broccoli, but which is better for us? We see discipline as something to chase against or an imposition to our happiness. Cultural messages and social acceptance hinge on following blind customs or our unhealthy, momentary decisions. We exercise our choice through making poor decisions. Freedom is confused with whim. An attempt to reign in stupidity is an act of aggression on society itself. Society has become such an entitled, precious bunch that the mere suggestion we tamp-down our instinctive responses feels like an insult. Where does that leave us?

If you think thumbing your nose at self-discipline will make you happier in the short or long-term, think again. In research, the higher a study subjected rated their self-control, the more satisfied they were in their lives. They were happier when they were faced with temptation. Similarly, other studies demonstrated that those who had strong self-control enjoyed closer relationships, as well as a more secure attachment within their relationships, lower rates of addiction, better performance at school, healthier emotional responses, and a higher self-esteem. But aren't those who have self-control beset with constant struggles against temptation? The research has demonstrated that with a good amount of self-control, people tend to minimize a situation that conflicts with their goals.

However, we can't always live in that stoic bubble. The movie theater example being the obvious reason. In those moments, however, you can acknowledge the unhealthy craving, desire, or bout of laziness; even respect it for a moment, as you reflect on its innate purpose within your primal history as a person. For example, the sugar used to be in limited supply, so sipping on soda was not even something a primal ancestor could fathom. You're able to understand it within the neurological and psychological aspects. And yet you can see it for what it is, an urge that doesn't deserve your interest, so treat it as such.

It's not about dampening your emotions when you feel drawn to dessert or appreciating the warm comfort of a bed when it's time to do a morning workout. It's about giving your inner backers what they're owed without classifying with the ones you don't want organizing your life. Controlling yourself isn't about controlling a particular self relative to your surroundings, but about dealing with your inner voices that are responding to it.

You can achieve this by practicing proper detachment, which is recognizing that something in you wants that cake rather than you wanting that cake. Rather than ignoring that confusing part of yourself, you can ask what else could take care of that part for the moment. Some people might require a little more care in that sense, and there is no judgement on that. It's all self-knowledge and useful to you.

Think about taking a long trip with kids. You pace the trip with their needs in mind. There are plenty of stops for potty breaks, well-timed snacks and meals to avoid grumpiness, a midday break that's longer for activities, and promises of pool time at the hotel. You provide them with the games, activities, and conversation you need to in order to keep them busy and happy during the long car ride. You have regard for their necessities as travelers with some limitations, but you don't relinquish the trip or ask them to drive the car for you.

You can attend to your inclinations and your sincere requirements behind them devoid of giving them ultimate rule over your life and well-being. You're tired at three in the afternoon? Walk away from the vending machine and go for a walk outside in the bright sunlight for a few minutes. If you work from home, take a fifteen minute power nap.

It's about learning to identify who you want leading your life. Your thoughts or the bigger awareness of your thoughts? You can call it self-control, maturity, or just willpower, but everyone has it. First you have to know that something or someone in you can actually do those actions. Many individuals never get to this point, deciding to fly by the following urge that comes about, flinging it into a huge mound that not once gives order to how they live their lives.

However, self-control isn't about what you give up, what you're saying no to, or what you're staying away from. It's what you're saying yes to, what is filing the space. If you focus your days on what you can't have, then you're still giving in to the power it's holding over you. You're still mentally obsessing about the cake even if you never ate a piece of it. At any moment, you can get perspective by asking yourself what you're mentally obsessing about.

What a lot easier is focusing on what you want to see happen, what you want to prioritize. You can either live in response to your environment or live with direction toward your life goals. True self-control isn't about restraint but about self-possession.

Self-control opens the door to intentional living for you. Your goals are next to impossible without having a little self-control. The fact is that self-control lets your intent have space that would otherwise be used by your momentary distractions and whims.

At self-control's best, it doesn't revolve around denial, deprivation, or chastising but intention, clarity, and attunement. You don't ignore these elements of yourself entirely, but become clear as to what role you want them to play in your decision-making process. You don't punish yourself or take pride in how little you can force yourself to live with. You make a bigger picture vision for your life and make choices that take care of your needs in ways that serve your plan.

In this way, self-control is the ultimate exercise of freedom.

Reflective Meditation

1. Sit comfortably and start by taking some slow and deep breaths to relax yourself.

2. When you feel fully relaxed, bring to mind a question you want to gain some deeper insight into. Say the question to yourself silently and slowly three times. Focus your attention on that question. You know you're grasping too tightly when your breathing increases and your body tenses. Relax and repeat.

3. Reflect on that question and explore its significant, meaning, and relationships to your life as deeply as possible.

4. When an insight surfaces, observe It without judgement. Hold it in your mind and feel it without emotion.

5. If you find you're losing focus, bring your attention back and repeat step two.

6. At the end of the session, write down any conclusions you've come to.

Chapter Seven - Accepting Life is a Finite Resource

Finally, you need to apply the final overlay. You can write about life as having an end, or you can think about it on a periodic basis. Step back from time to time and really allow it to sink that everything in your life is simply a loan. That means that everything, your partner, children, parents, friends, work, possessions, property, joy, talents, and awe, are borrowed. You get to play for a while, and then it's all gone.

Some will choose to attach a religious meaning to this idea. Some choose to believe that this idea stands on its own without a religious connotation. The point is the same no matter what. You take in the fact that life existed before you and it will exist after you're gone. Everyone you love will come to the same end.

Some might file this under religion, and others might view this as a connection to the ongoing nature of life, or even the laws of evolution. This is the heart of the stoic perspective itself. It's about being at the center of our lives, but not about manhandling life or detaching entirely from it, but to live deliberately and lightly at the same time. When you mind your time and thoughts well, you can better enjoy the adventures that are to come.

Quotes about Death

You are younger; but what does that matter? There is no fixed count of our years. You do not know where death awaits you; so be ready for it everywhere. ~ Seneca

When Seneca said this, he meant to bring attention to the fact that you should never assume that you will live another day. For many, this means that you should never procrastinate, go to bed without saying you love someone who means a lot to you, or take for granted their kindness in return. We take everything for granted, assuming that it will be there tomorrow. However, many of us have seen enough to curb this thought pattern because tomorrow is not guaranteed to be there.

That doesn't mean you should go about life living every day as if it's your last because that would mean never going to work, never planning ahead, and never looking to the future. However, it does mean you shouldn't put off the things you really want to do in life. Don't think you'll be able to go skiing all of your retirement years because you might not make it that long. Make some plans to go skiing and enjoy life when you have a little vacation time. Don't have vacation time? Make some.

"What?" I say to myself; "does death so often test me? Let it do so; I myself have for a long time tested death." "When?" you ask. Before I was born. Death is non-existence, and I know already what that means. What was before me will happen again after me. If there is any suffering in this state, there must have been such suffering also in the past, before we entered the light of day. As a matter of fact, however, we felt no discomfort then. And I ask you, would you not say that one was the greatest of fools who believed that a lamp was worse off when it was extinguished than before it was lighted? We mortals also are lighted and extinguished; the period of suffering comes in between, but on either side there is a deep peace. For, unless I am very much mistaken, my dear Lucilius, we go astray in thinking that death only follows, when in reality it has both preceded us and will in turn follow us. Whatever condition existed before our birth, is death. For what does it matter whether you do not begin at all, or whether you leave off, inasmuch as the result of both these states is non-existence? ~ Seneca

This is a long passage, but it explains the very essence of a stoic's viewpoint on death. There was 'nothingness' before we were born, and there will be 'nothingness' after we are dead. At both points, we're non-existent to the world. Between birth and death, we live lives full of peaks, valleys, suffering, and happiness. We're lighted and extinguished with serenity on both sides.

There are times when we ought to die and are unwilling; sometimes we die and are unwilling. No one is so ignorant as not to know that we must at some time die; nevertheless, when one draws near death, one turns to flight, trembles, and laments. Would you not think him an utter fool who wept because he was not alive a thousand years ago? And is he not just as much of a fool who weeps because he will not be alive a thousand years from now? It is all the same; you will not be, and you were not. Neither of these periods of time belongs to you. You have been cast upon this point of time; if you would make it longer, how much longer shall you make it? Why weep? Why pray? You are taking pains to no purpose. ~ Seneca

In this paragraph, Seneca is calling out to those who are worried about dying and letting them know that neither of these moments are ones you can control. You can't choose when you die, just as you can't choose to be born later or earlier in time. The only time you have control over is the time in which you're alive – the here and now.

Don't worry about the past or future, but be focused on the present. Make plans for the future to achieve your goals and strive for your greatest moments of happiness with each decision you make.

And, on the other hand, if death comes near with its summons, even though it be untimely in its arrival, though it cut one off in one's prime, a man has had a taste of all that the longest life can give. Such a man has in great measure come to understand the universe. He knows that honorable things do not depend on time for their growth; but any life must seem short to those who measure its length by pleasures which are empty and for that reason unbounded. ~ Seneca

In this passage, Seneca is being brutally honest. Our lives shouldn't be judged by length but by our achievements. We should live with purpose and not give in to the easy temptations. We're surrounded by people who are unhappy because they have no sense of purpose.

Debt, obesity, and mental gluttony are a common sight. It's easy to fall pretty to being lazy, but be mindful that your existence is not forever. You only get one chance at this thing known as life. Live it to your fullest capabilities.

'Time goes,' but 'Time flies,' because the latter is the quickest kind of movement, and in every case our best days are the first to be snatched away; why, then, do we hesitate to bestir ourselves so that we may be able to keep pace with this swiftest of all swift things?" The good flies past and the bad takes its place. Just as the purest wine flows from the top of the jar and the thickest dregs settle at the bottom; so in our human life, that which is best comes first. Shall we allow other men to quaff the best, and keep the dregs for ourselves? ~ Seneca

In this passage, Seneca is musing about how many people waste away their best years of their lives for someone else when they could be spending them on themselves. People who are in their prime are living boring, routine lives as they try to make as much money as possible or they try to climb the corporate ladder. As Seneca says, the good flies past.

It's a crime to waste away your better years. Your finest years are swiftly behind you and you're left with nothing but improbability in the future. Health problems will crop before you even feel 'old'. In the United States in 2014, 585000+ individuals passed from cancer. Go a few years before and none of those people most likely saw their death coming. It's never known when you'll die, so don't waste your younger years, and don't think that the years in your fifties and sixties are not younger because you may find yourself in your nineties in no time.

Because in our youth we are able to learn; we can bend to nobler purposes minds that are ready and still pliable; because this is the time for work, the time for keeping our minds busied in study and in exercising our bodies with useful effort; for that which remains is more sluggish and lacking in spirit — nearer the end. ~ Seneca

In this passage, Seneca is saying that we should take risks and work hard when we're young and healthy. That is the time to experiment and find out what we love, where we want to be, and who we want to spend time with. We should be working out and reading on a daily basis. Ignorance isn't an excuse at this point in our lives.

It is low and mean to live in the usual and conventional way. Let us abandon the ordinary sort of day. Let us have a morning that is a special feature of ours, peculiar to ourselves!" Such men are, in my opinion, as good as dead. Are they not all but present at a funeral —and before their time too —when they live amid torches and tapers? ~ Seneca

In this paragraph about death, Seneca is looking down upon those who choose to live an ordinary life. Following the societal norms is safe and easy. Seneca is calling these people as good as dead. Straying from the path is unknown and dangerous, so many people don't try to attempt an extraordinary feat. Original thought is no longer something to be proud of, and conformity is the expected of the people because it ensures survival of the current societal hierarchy.

Our span of life is divided into parts; it consists of large circles enclosing smaller. One circle embraces and bounds the rest; it reaches from birth to the last day of existence. The next circle limits the period of our young manhood. The third confines all of childhood in its circumference. Again, there is, in a class by itself, the year; it contains within itself all the divisions of time by the multiplication of which we get the total of life. The month is bounded by a narrower ring. The smallest circle of all is the day; but even a day has its beginning and its ending, its sunrise and its sunset. ~ Seneca

Seneca is breaking down life into a series of stages in this section. He's saying that we're born and we die, and that is the circle of life. Smaller circles within that one can include the years, months, and days we live. Most of us like to use years as our life's compass. Rather than doing that, try to estimate your remaining life in days, minutes, and seconds. It gives you a different perspective on things and makes you view life with a great appreciation.

Stoicism teaches you that you should only fear what you can control. Seneca's words about death are comforting and the perspective is logical. Death isn't something we're able to control. It'll happen one day, maybe sooner rather than later, but we don't know when. Therefore, thinking about your demise is a poor use of your life.

Thoughts about death are crippling, as are other damaging emotions like anger, greed, and jealousy. It's up to you to create a strong mindset and learn self-control. Be with your body and mind, and you'll never fall victim to your irrational thoughts.

Yes, thoughts of death will come to you from time to time, but try not to dwell on them for too long. Live your life, be mindful of where you are now, and aim for great things in the future.

Conclusion

As a conclusion, I'd like to talk about some of the benefits of Stoicism and how it's helped others in the past. While there are many applicable steps in this book, sometimes it's better to understand *why* you're doing something rather than just blindly following a faith or belief system, and Stoicism is a way of life or a belief system.

Stoicism Helps You Remain Calm and Collected in the Face of Adversity

People often see stoics as emotional drones who never feel anything, but stoics feel just as much as the next person. The difference is they're able to remain calm during a terrible situation. A stoic is the person who is able to logically think their way out of a tricky situation, and when they can't, they take the consequences of that situation with dignity. It means they understand and accept their fate, and they are able to say they've lived life to its fullest.

For example, if one of your children breaks a leg, it does no good to run around the yard screaming about the situation. It's better for your child and you if you're able to keep a calm façade and drive your child to the nearest emergency center. Crying, screaming, and swerving through traffic only causes your child and you more stress, and potentially, more danger. A stoic is able to handle the situation and the bad emotions that come with it.

Stoicism Helps You Make Better Decisions

Being a stoic is about thinking. Seneca, Aurelius, and many other infamous stoics were infamous because they thought long and hard about decisions and life. Rather than being impulsive and eating an entire cake, you'll think about your desires and eat a more appropriate slice of cake. Instead of taking that leap off a second-story roof into a pool, you'll think about the consequences if you miss the pool before you act.

In a way, stoicism teaches you to be a more logical thinker without sacrificing your happiness and joy. You can still do the things that make you happy, but you do them in a safer, more constructive way.

Stoicism Teaches You Failure is Something to Learn From

Everyone fails, and stoicism helps you take that failure with dignity, as well as helps you pick up and move forward in life while learning your lesson. When you take time to be in the present moment, think about your failure, and realize how you may have prevented it, then you've learned something about yourself and what you were attempting to do. If you dwell on the negative emotions of failure and never take a look at *why* you failed, then you won't learn.

However, stoicism also teaches us that failure is a part of life. It's something that will happen to everyone, and has happened to everyone. No one walks for the first time without falling. No one speaks their first word without first babbling as an infant. We're all made up of our failures, and stoicism teaches us that it's alright to fail, and to move forward with our lives.